First Aid

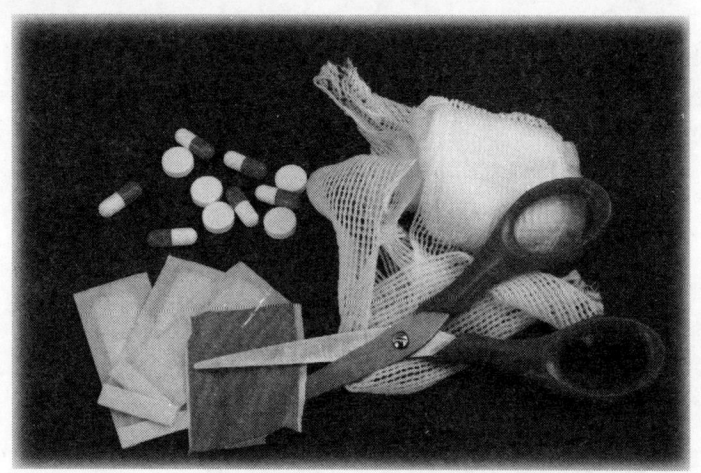

Health Solutions
First Aid

Edited by
Dr Savitri Ramaiah

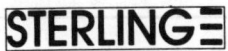

STERLING PAPERBACKS
An imprint of
Sterling Publishers (P) Ltd.
Regd. Office: A1/256 Safdarjung Enclave,
New Delhi-110029. CIN: U22110DL1964PTC211907
Tel: 26387070, 26386209; Fax: 91-11-26383788
E-mail: mail@sterlingpublishers.in
www.sterlingpublishers.in

Health Solutions First Aid
© 2019, Sterling Publishers Private Limited
ISBN 978 81 207 3328 2
First Edition 2008
Reprint 2010, 2011, 2015

All rights are reserved. No part of this publication may be reproduced, stored in a retrieval system or transmitted, in any form or by any means, mechanical, photocopying, recording or otherwise, without prior written permission of the publisher.

PRINTED IN INDIA

Printed and Published by Sterling Publishers Pvt. Ltd.,
Plot No. 13, Ecotech-III, Greater Noida - 201306, Uttar Pradesh, India

Information for this series, has been provided by *Health Update*, a monthly bulletin of the Society for Health Education and Learning Packages. The Update is intended to provide you with knowledge to adopt preventive measures and cooperate with the doctor during illness for better outcome of treatment.

Contributor

 Nature Cure
Dr Dara Amar
(Prof. and Head, Department of Community Medicine, St. John's Medical College, Bangalore)

Preface

Health Solutions is an easy-to-read reference series put together by *Health Update* and assisted by a team of medical experts who offer the latest perspectives on body health.

Each book in the series enhances your knowledge on a particular health issue. It makes you an active participant by giving multiple perspectives to choose from.

This book is intended as a home adviser but does not substitute a doctor.

The opinions are those of the contributors, and the publisher holds no responsibility.

Contents

Preface	7
Introduction	11
How should the clothing be removed?	15
What is the First Aid for suffocation?	16
How is artificial respiration given?	19
How is external heart massage given?	22
How should an affected person be carried?	25
How should a person with injuries to the neck and backbone be carried?	34
What is the First Aid for bleeding injuries?	37
What is the First Aid for burns?	41
What is the First Aid for animal bites?	49
What is the First Aid for poison?	53
What is the First Aid for wounds during children's play and accidental falls by adults?	56

What is the First Aid for a cramp?	60
What is the First Aid for winding?	62
What is the First Aid for stitch?	63
What is the First Aid for heat stroke?	64
What is the First Aid for fainting?	66
What is the First Aid for a fracture?	71

Introduction

First Aid is the treatment given to a person before a doctor arrives.

The main objectives of first aid are:
- To preserve life.
- To promote recovery.
- To prevent worsening of the condition.
- To take the injured to a safer place where professionals can look after them.

First Aid can be done by anybody and anywhere but one should be aware of first aid methods for specific situations.

This book tells you how to approach the affected person and what to do before beginning specific procedures.

The methods of First Aid had begun to evolve ever since one human desired to help another in pain. In fact this instinctive and instant behaviour to protect one's own was part of the survival strategy. The behaviour patterns to protect others got repeated and passed on to others as learned

behaviours. These ranged from simple tasks such as removing a thorn to pressing one's hand against an animal inflicted wound to stop the bleeding during a hunt for food. These protective acts were performed by almost everybody and had four main purposes. These included:
- to preserve life,
- to promote recovery,
- to prevent worsening of the condition and
- finally to carry away the injured to a safer place where more experienced healers could look after them.

The earlier the protective acts were accomplished, the better were the chances of survival and recovery. People paid first attention to signs of difficult breathing, bleeding and unconsciousness in order to prevent death. Thus, the familiar "immediate attention and action" that needed to be done then and there by anybody and everybody before rushing the injured to more experienced healers, became the basic principle and aim of what came to be formally known as First Aid.

By its very nature and meaning, First Aid can be done anywhere and everywhere and by everyone. Situations where First Aid becomes necessary can vary from factory sites, road injuries, farming areas, jungles and deserts, building collapses, fire breakouts, floods and drowning, animal and plant poisonings and finally, our own homes.

Box 1: Approach to First Aid

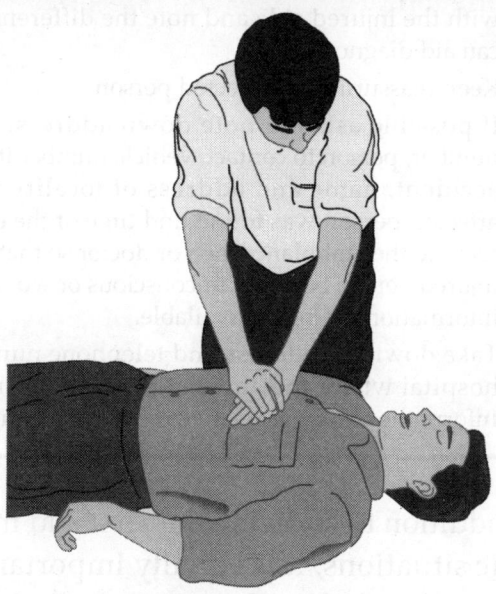

1. First check for breathing and apply artificial respiration if needed.
2. Check for the heartbeat and apply external heart massage, if needed.
3. Control bleeding, if any.
4. If the environment is dangerous because of fire, building collapse, etc., move the affected person to a safety zone. Be careful in case of back injuries that may affect the spine.
5. Request for control and dispersal of the crowds in order to give air and space for first aid procedures.
6. Send for a doctor.
7. For helping in the diagnosis and treatment of poisoning, preserve any bottles of chemicals, drugs, etc., found near the affected person.

> 8. Examine the affected person thoroughly while waiting for transportation. Compare the normal side of the body with the injured side and note the differences as they can aid diagnosis.
> 9. Keep reassuring the affected person.
> 10. If possible ask and note down address, telephone number, person to contact, vehicle number if there is an accident, name and address of locality where the affected person was found and time of the event. Give these to the ambulance men or doctor so that in case the injured person becomes unconscious or worse, this vital information is already available.
> 11. Take down the address and telephone number of the hospital where the affected person is being shifted. Inform the family or relatives or friends immediately.

In addition to knowing the First Aid methods for specific situations, it is equally important to know how to approach the affected person and what to do before beginning specific procedures. Box 1 lists the approach to First Aid.

How should the clothing be removed?

This is always a delicate issue especially if the affected person is in a public place. Do not err on the side of excessive modesty nor go to the other extreme of immediately stripping the patient in the name of giving urgent First Aid.

Expose only the injured parts for immediate treatment. In case of loosening clothes to aid breathing, do just that but do not expose the body too much as it may result in symptoms of shock if exposed to the cool air, especially in case of bleeding.

If necessary, slit the sleeves of shirts and coats covering the affected limb. Do this preferably along the seams so that the coat or shirt can be repaired later. You can also slit trousers in the same way, if necessary.

In the case of boots or shoes, cut the laces to aid fast removal as time is important in giving First Aid.

Socks are difficult to remove without painful manipulation. You can slit them by inserting two fingers between the sock and the leg and cutting between your fingers.

What is the First Aid for suffocation?

In case of suffocation, any delay in action can result in permanent brain damage even if the person is ultimately saved. Speed is essential. Signs of suffocation include:
- Rapid but shallow breathing, often with gasps in between;
- The lips, nails, fingers, toes and face begin to turn blue;
- Veins in the neck may begin to swell; and
- Pulse will become rapid but hardly detectable.

Steps for providing First Aid in case of suffocation include the following:

1. Remove the cause of suffocation. It could be either food, water, foreign body, gas in the air passage. Sometimes the tongue falls back in an unconscious person which results in strangulation. So one should try and remove the obstruction. The same applies in the case of

hanging, smothering, electric shock, crush injuries, etc.
2. Place the affected person on his/her back.
3. Support the back of the neck with one hand and use your other hand to press back the head towards the ground. This will make the air passage straight.
4. Get somebody to tightly roll a small towel and place it under the neck (not head) where your hand was acting as a support so far. This will free your hands to proceed with artificial respiration.
5. Give artificial respiration whenever there is slight but difficult breathing.
6. Check for the pulse by feeling it with two fingers inserted between the lower end of the voice box (Adam's apple) and the neck muscle adjacent to it. The pulse at the wrist is not dependable in such cases.
7. If the pulse is felt, then proceed with artificial respiration.
8. Do not stop artificial respiration until well after normal and spontaneous breathing has been resumed since the brain can be damaged due to lack of oxygen.
9. If the pulse is also not felt, you need to combine external heart massage with artificial respiration. It is important to remember that people

providing First Aid are better at this situation than just anyone. The ratio of artificial respiration to heart massage should be 2:15. This means that two lung expansions are necessary for fifteen heart massages.
10. Keep the airways are clear and if obstructed, use the technique to remove foreign bodies from the throat.

How is artificial respiration given?

Although many methods of artificial respiration have been evolved, the most effective is the mouth-to-mouth method. Steps involved in providing mouth-to-mouth respiration include the following:

1. Keep the affected person on his/her back and place a rolled up towel under his/her neck. This will extend the neck straight and tilt the head backwards.
2. Sit on the right side of the affected person and use your left hand thumb and forefinger to pinch his/her nostrils shut.
3 Such a posture will prevent the air from escaping out of his/her nose instead of going into his/her lung when you blow down into the mouth.
4. Place your right hand thumb on the affected person's chin and pull down his/her lower jaw to keep the mouth open.

5. Take a deep breath now with your mouth fully open. Then, clamp down your open mouth on to the affected person's open mouth and blow down hard enough to make his/her chest wall rise.
6. Ensure that your open mouth covers the affected person's mouth smugly so that there is no chance for leakage of air while you blow down.
7. Withdraw your mouth and watch the affected person's chest wall fall back on its own.

At the end of the above steps, you complete one cycle of breathing for the affected person. Repeat this continuously at the rate of fifteen to twenty times per minute. You can use a thin handkerchief to cover the affected person's mouth for hygienic purposes, before you blow down. In the case of children, your mouth can cover its nose and mouth without pinching the nose and blow gently.

You may also use mouth-to-nose method but then keep the affected person's mouth shut with your right hand.

The two stages of mouth-to-mouth respiration are as illustrated in Figure 1.

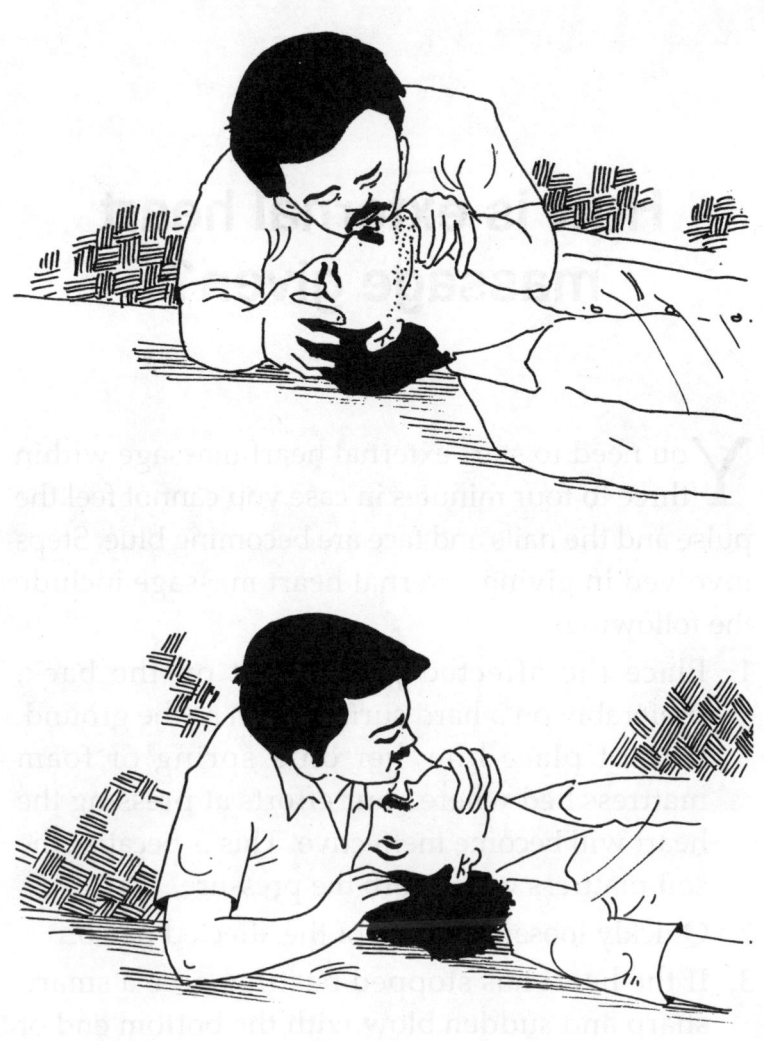

Figure 1: Stages of mouth-to-mouth respiration

How is external heart massage given?

You need to start external heart massage within three to four minutes in case you cannot feel the pulse and the nails and face are becoming blue. Steps involved in giving external heart massage include the following:

1. Place the affected person flat on the back, preferably on a hard surface such as the ground. Do not place him/her on a spring or foam mattress bed where your efforts at pressing the heart will become ineffective. This is because the soft mattress will absorb the pressure.
2. Quickly loosen clothing of the affected person.
3. If the heart has stopped beating, give a smart, sharp and sudden blow with the bottom end of your tightly clenched fist on the lower and left side of the breast bone.
4. Use one stroke per second for about ten to fifteen seconds. Always feel if the pulse has restarted, at the root of the neck between the lower end of the

voice box or wind-pipe and the adjacent neck muscle. If this does not start the heartbeat, immediately proceed to the next steps.

5. Kneel down to the right side (left side if simultaneous artificial respiration is going on) of the affected person.
6. Bend over and place the heel of your hand on the lower part of the breast-bone. Next, place the heel of your other hand over and across your first hand as shown in Figure 2. The fingers of both your hands must be free and not touch the affected person's chest. It is important to remember that the heel of your hand is the sturdiest part of your hand.

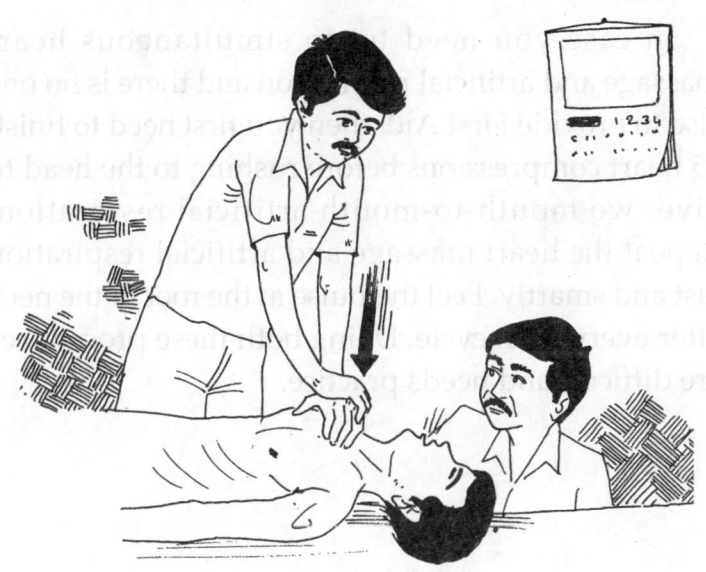

Figure 2: External heart massage

7. Press down firmly on the breast-bone with your hands in a rhythmic manner at the rate of sixty presses per minute in adults.
8. In small children, you can use the heel of only one hand but press down eighty to ninety times per minute. Do not press so forcefully that the ribs crack.
9. In the case of hand-held babies up to two years, use only two fingers at about hundred presses per minute. The frequencies of pressures applied correspond to their respective heartbeats per minute.
10. Continue till pulse returns and still further thereafter till pink colour returns to nails and face.

In case you need to do simultaneous heart massage and artificial respiration and there is no one else to provide First Aid, then you first need to finish 15 heart compressions before rushing to the head to give two mouth-to-mouth artificial respiration. Repeat the heart massage and artificial respiration fast and smartly. Feel the pulse at the root of the neck after every such cycle. Doing both these procedures are difficult and needs practice.

How should an affected person be carried?

Often the main problem at the site of accident, etc., is how to carry the affected person. People believe that carrying a person is a natural thing to do and does not require specific procedures.

This is however not always true. If the recommended guidelines for carrying an affected person are not followed, it may either add to the injuries already sustained or aggravate them.

When there is only **one person to provide First Aid**, the following procedures are recommended:

Cradle method

This method involves carrying the affected person, especially children, by supporting your left arm under the affected person's bent knees while your right arm supports the neck. It is important to remember that this method of carrying the injured is recommended only for minor injuries. It should not be performed when injury to the backbone is suspected.

Human crutch method

This method is recommended when there is injury to only one upper limb and the affected person is conscious and he/she is able to walk with assistance. To provide such assistance, position yourself at his/her uninjured side. Help him/her to walk by putting one of your arms around his/her waist and holding on to his/her hip clothing. Place the affected person's uninjured hand around your neck and use your other free arm to hold it as shown in Figure 3.

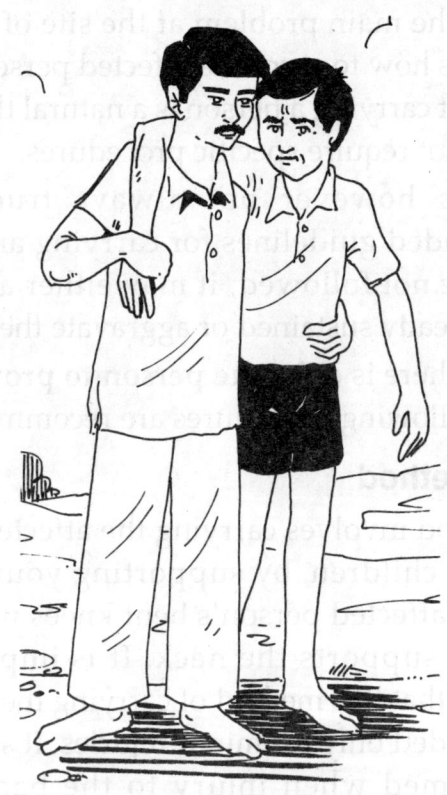

Figure 3: Human crutch

Piggy-back method

If the affected person is unable to walk but is conscious, then you can carry him/her "piggyback", i.e., on your back. Help the affected person get on to your back and ask him/her to hold you by embracing you from behind. Bring both his/her legs forward on either side of your waist and support his/her legs under the knees.

Fireman's lift

This method is used only if you think you can bear the full weight of the affected person. This manoeuvre requires you to be physically strong and is done when the affected person is unconscious and you are alone. Steps involved in Fireman's lift include the following:

- Support the affected person with both hands and your body. Pull him/her to an upright position against the wall.
- Lean and support against the affected person, using your right side of your body.
- Grasp his/her right wrist with your left hand and lift it.
- Bend down slowly and put your head under his/her extended right arm so that your right shoulder is level with the lower part of his/her abdomen.
- Place your free right arm between his/her thighs.

- Take the affected person's entire weight on your right shoulder and at the same time slowly but strongly rise to an erect standing position.
- Quickly adjust and pull the affected person across both your shoulders and balance his/her weight equally across the shoulders.
- Transfer the affected person's right wrist to your right hand. This will free your left hand, which you may use to hold onto railings of a staircase or even the side of a ladder as you perhaps descend from an upstairs room, etc.

Fireman's method is shown in Figure 4.

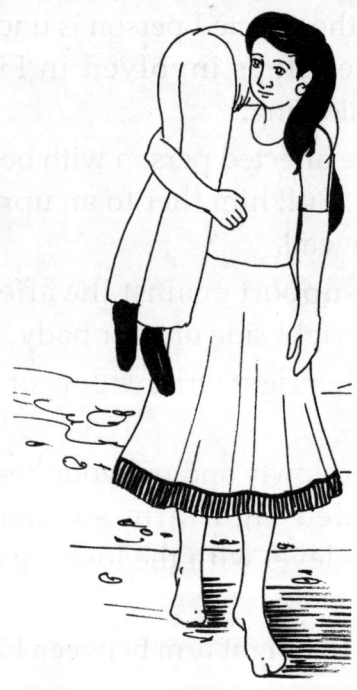

Figure 4: Fireman's lift

When there are **two persons to provide First Aid**, the following procedures are recommended:

Four-hand seat

This is recommended if the affected person is conscious but is unable to walk. Steps involved in making the four-hand seat include the following:

- Face the other person providing First Aid behind the affected person.
- Approach each other and grasp each other's right wrist with your left hand. This forms a square shaped four-hand seat as shown in Figure 5.
- Both of you then need to grasp your own left wrist with your own right hand.

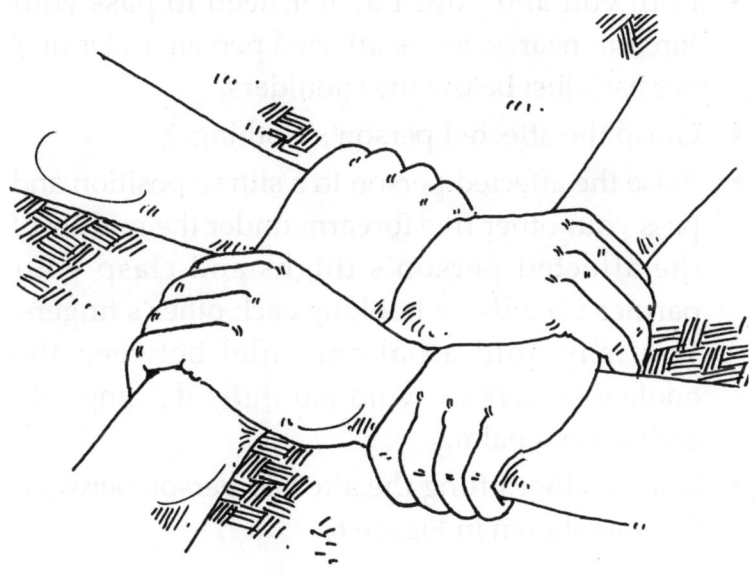

Figure 5: Four-hand seat

- Instruct the affected person to put one arm around you and your partner to steady himself/herself and sit on the four-hand seat.
- Your partner and you can now carry the affected person by walking normally.

Two-hand seat

This method is recommended if the affected person is not able to assist you by putting his/her arms around you and your partner. Steps involved in making a two-hand seat include the following:
- Make the affected person lie down on the back.
- Face the other person providing First Aid and bend down on each side of the affected person.
- Both you and your partner need to pass your forearm nearest to the affected person under his/her back just below the shoulders.
- Grasp the affected person's clothing.
- Raise the affected person to a sitting position and pass your other free forearm under the middle of the affected person's thighs and clasp your partner's hands by hooking each other's fingers. You may hold a handkerchief between the hooked fingers to avoid painfully digging into each other's palm.
- Rise together lifting the affected person between them as shown in Figure 6.

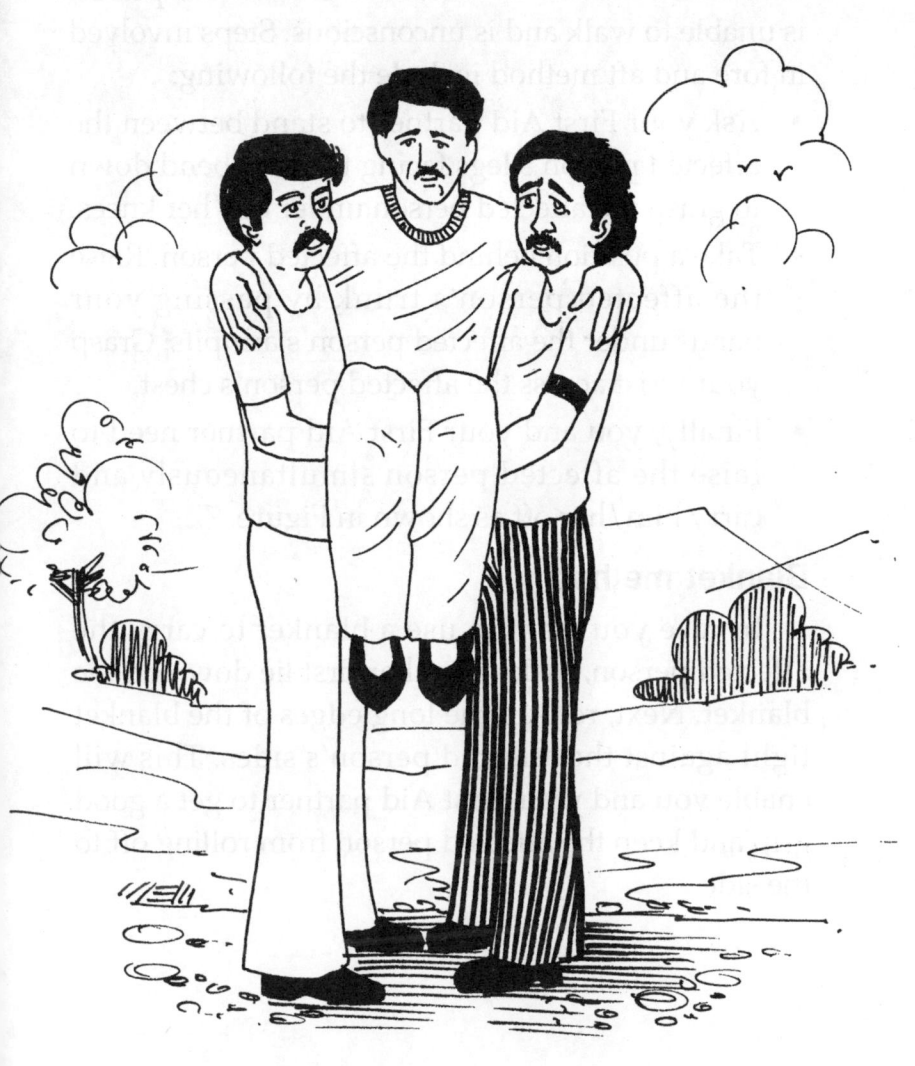

Figure 6: Two-hand seat

Fore and aft method

This method is recommended if the affected person is unable to walk and is unconscious. Steps involved in fore and aft method include the following:

- Ask your First Aid partner to stand between the affected person's legs facing the feet, bend down to grasp the affected person under his/her knees.
- Take a position behind the affected person. Raise the affected person's trunk by passing your hands under the affected person's armpits. Grasp your wrist across the affected person's chest.
- Finally, you and your First Aid partner need to raise the affected person simultaneously and carry him/her off as shown in Figure 7.

Blanket method

In case you want to use a blanket to carry the affected person, make him/her first lie down on the blanket. Next, roll-up the long edges of the blanket tight against the affected person's sides. This will enable you and your First Aid partner to get a good grip and keep the affected person from rolling off to the side.

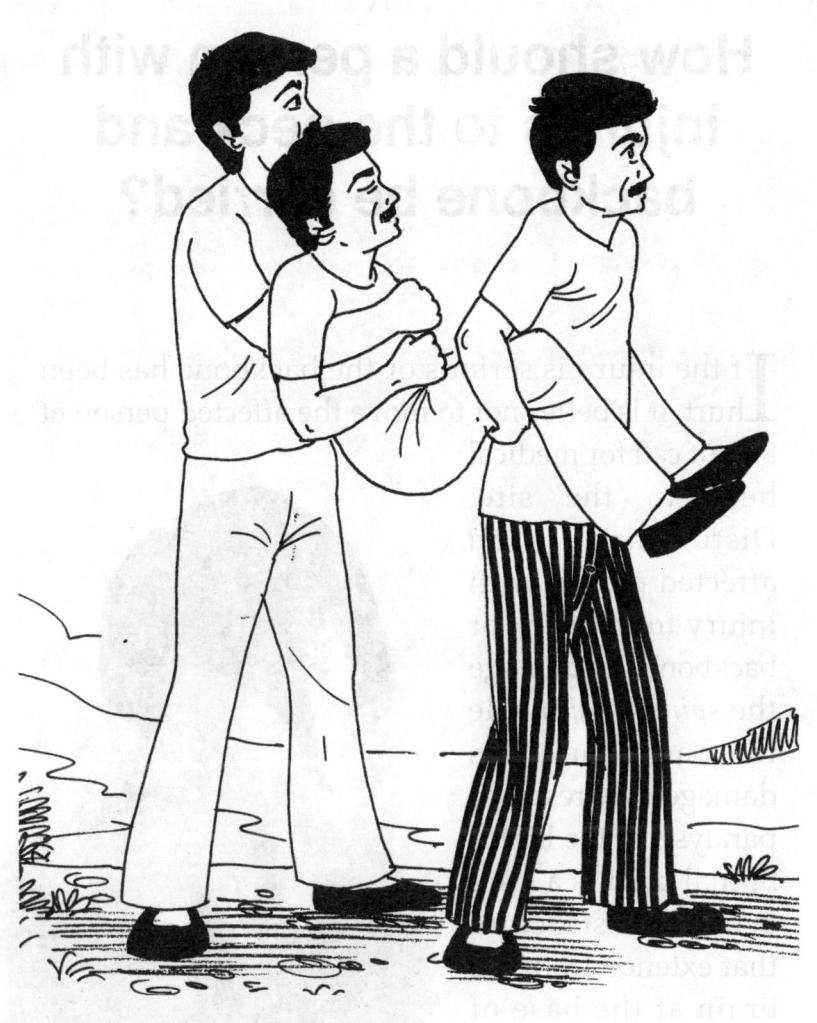

Figure 7: Fore and aft method

How should a person with injuries to the neck and backbone be carried?

If the injury is serious or the backbone has been hurt, it is better not to move the affected person at all but call for medical help to the site. Disturbing an affected person with injury to the neck or backbone can damage the *spinal cord* inside the backbone. This damage may result in paralysis of the limbs. Spinal cord is a long cylindrical structure that extends from the brain at the base of the skull to the back. It is a major part of the

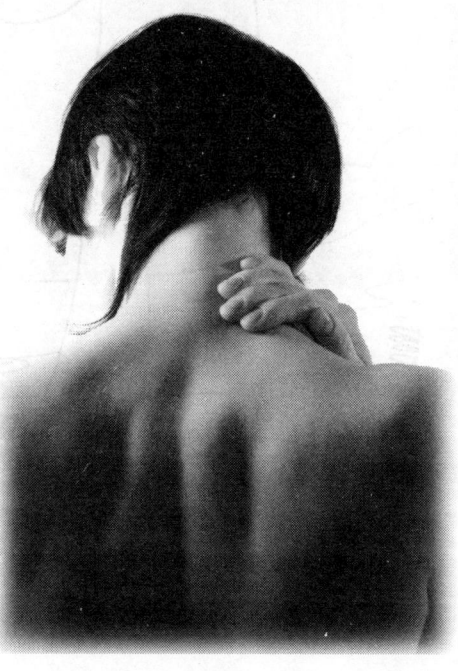

central nervous system and carries impulses to and from the brain.

- For all back injuries, do not allow affected person to move. Keep him/her still.
- Carefully, place pads of towel between the affected person's thighs, knees and ankles and then tie the limbs with broad bandages or cloth at the thighs, knees and ankles.
- Transport him/her by a stretcher or a sufficiently broad board of wood. Always keep the affected person's face upwards for least damage to the backbone.
- The main aim of First Aid in case of injuries to the neck or backbone is to give equal and coordinated support to the head, neck, back, thighs and ankles and keep the affected person's body in a straight line without disturbing the trunk. These measures can protect the spinal cord inside the backbone.
- At least four First Aid people are needed to support the affected person with both hands, making sure that there are no jerks.
- The first person needs to support the head and neck, the second person the back, the third person the thighs and the fourth person the leg and ankles.
- Lift the affected person while keeping the body straight as high as the surface of the stretcher and slip the stretcher under him/her.

- In case of neck injuries, make sure that the breathing is not affected.
- It is important to remember that you need to carry the stretcher slowly.
- You may bind the affected person to the stretcher at the hips and thighs to prevent unnecessary rolling.

What is the First Aid for bleeding injuries?

In small cuts or pricks, the bleeding usually stops by itself through a clotting mechanism. However, in case of deep cut injuries, the bleeding can occur from arteries or veins.

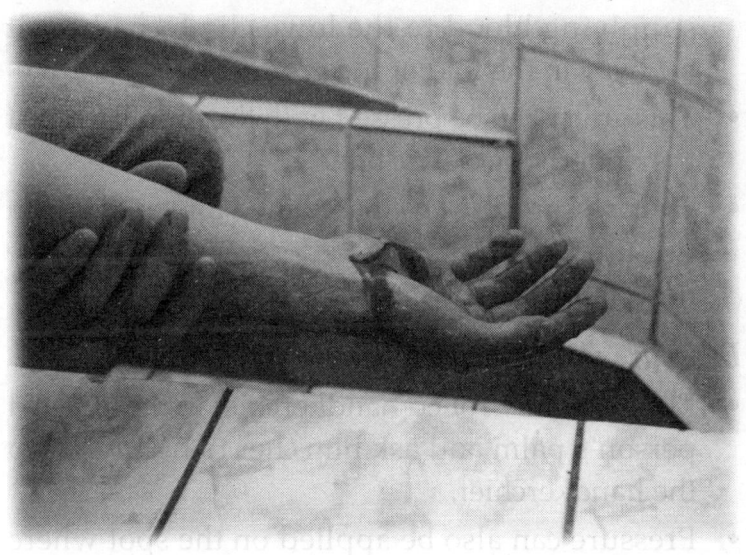

In the case of arteries, the blood comes out in jets (corresponding with the beat of the heart) and its colour will be bright red.

In case there is bleeding from the artery, press firmly a clean pad made of washed handkerchief at the site of bleeding in order to stop it immediately. If bleeding continues do not take off the original pad but add more similar pads.

You can also stop bleeding by pressing on certain pressure points depending on where the bleeding occurs. Ultimately, however, the affected person must be taken to the hospital. The most common pressure points are:

Pressure point for the thighs and below:
- Bend the knees slightly. The main artery supplying blood to the lower limb can be felt midway in the fold of the groin.
- This artery can be pressed with the thumb against the underlying pelvic bone.
- The pressure must be maintained for ten to fifteen minutes until the affected person reaches the hospital.

Pressure point for the palm and fingers:
- Place a tightly rolled handkerchief in the affected person's palm and ask him/her to tightly grasp the handkerchief.
- Pressure can also be applied on the spot where the pulse of a person is normally felt.

Pressure point for upper limb:
- The main artery supplying the upper limb runs along the inner border of the biceps muscle.
- Apply pressure on the inner side of the middle of the upper arm and press the artery against the underlying bone.

Pressure point for the face:
- Apply pressure on the artery that can be felt along the lower border of the lower jaw, just in front of the lower jaw angle.

Pressure point for the side of the head:
- Apply pressure about an inch in front of the upper part of the ear.

Bleeding from the nose:
- Ask the patient to breathe through the mouth and to bend the head forward.
- Pinch the soft part of the nostrils together firmly until the bleeding stops.
- Next, place a cold compress consisting of broken ice cubes in a handkerchief across the nose for ten minutes.

Bleeding from gums:
- Rinse the mouth with diluted salt water.
- Place a thick cotton ball against the bleeding gum and ask the patient to bite on the cotton ball until the bleeding subsides.

Bleeding from the scalp:
- The bleeding from the scalp can look very alarming because of the large number of superficial veins.
- To stop the bleeding, apply a large pad and a bandage against the bleeding area.
- Consult with a doctor to rule out possible internal head injuries.
- You also need to monitor the patient's level of consciousness.

What is the First Aid for burns?

The danger of burns depends on the area of burns rather than the degree or depth of the burn. Guidelines for First Aid for burns are as listed below:
- Use plain water freely not only to quench the fire but also to cool the burnt area rapidly so that skin damage is minimised.
- Do not use ice cold water as the ice may intensify the shock reaction of the patient.
- Do not allow the patient to run.
- Do not open doors and windows to allow fresh air in as it only makes the fire burn more intensively.
- While approaching the patient it is advisable to hold a thick rug or blanket, in front of you and immediately wrap the burning patient in it.
- The patient must be made to lie down quickly and the flames smothered by gentle rolling or gentle pats on the flames with the rug, etc.

- Do not use thin fabrics or plastic or synthetic materials for putting out the flames.
- While rescuing persons from a burning room, remember that fresh air is available at ground level. Therefore, you must crawl along the floor to pull out the patient.
- However, do not crawl in case of LPG fires since gas is heavier than air and sinks to the floor level.
- Always wear a wet handkerchief round your face when going to rescue from fire.
- Carbon monoxide may be present if wood fires, car exhausts in car sheds, charcoal fires are present. In such cases, speed of rescue is important for both, you and the affected person.
- Do not try to remove sticking particles of charred clothing from the patient's body.
- Cover the burnt area with clean and dry cloth.
- Do not apply any oil, ointments or lotions at home since this may carry infection.
- Remove rings, bangles, belts and shoes immediately as it would be difficult to remove them later when the limbs begin to swell.
- Transport affected person immediately to the hospital.

For minor burns and scalds due to boiling water:
- Submerge the burnt area immediately in cold water (not ice water).

- Cover the burn with a clean dry cloth but not cotton as it will stick in the wound and become painful to remove later.
- Do not open blisters as this can cause infection and scarring.
- Do not apply any oils as they may lead to infection later.

In case of chemical burns:
- Wash the area with large amounts of water in order to reduce damage.
- In the case of chemical burns to eyes, make the patient lie down.
- Keep the eye open and pour water into the eyes from the inner corner of the eye outwardly to prevent the other eye from being affected.
- Do not allow patient to rub the eyes.
- In case of children, tie their hands behind the back to prevent rubbing the eyes.
- Cover the affected eye and seek medical help immediately.

In case of electric shock
- It is important to remember that a higher current causes more damage than a higher voltage.
- While every effort must be made to instantly switch off the source of electricity, time should not be wasted while removing the patient from the electrical source.

- Push the patient with any wooden, plastic materials or a dry rope or even a hastily removed shirt or any other clothing material.
- There should be no metal. Do not use metal knives or scissors to cut the wires.
- Water and oil are dangerous conductors of electricity.
- If in shock or suffering from electrical burns, transfer the affected person immediately to a hospital.
- Burns by electrical shock can be extremely painful, as they are deep burns.

Foreign body in the eye:
- The cardinal rule is to never rub the eye. In case of children, tie their hands at the back to prevent rubbing.
- Penetrating foreign bodies with bleeding and imbedded foreign bodies in the black of the eye (cornea) require immediate medical attention.
- In such cases, even the other normal eye may undergo what is called as a *sympathetic reaction* and blindness may follow.
- If the foreign body is visible under the eyelids, remove it carefully with the corner of a clean handkerchief twisted to a fine point as shown in Figure 8.
- In the case of the upper eyelid, turn up the lid to spot the foreign body, then remove it. This requires skill.

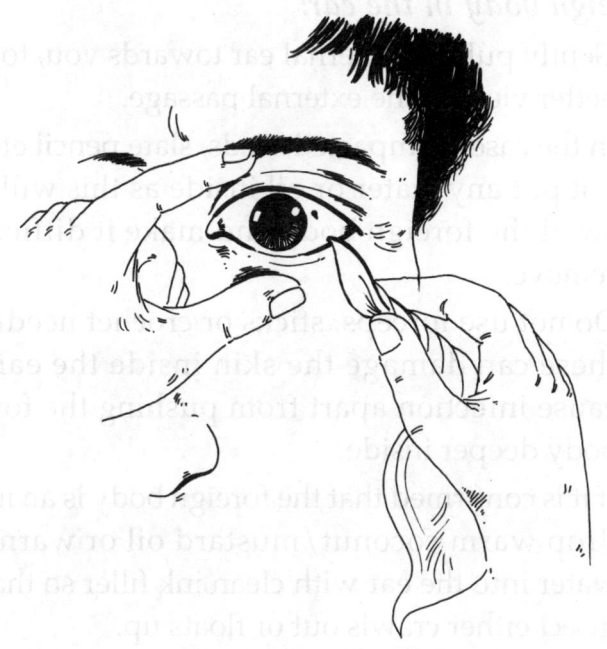

Figure 8: Removing foreign body from the eye

- Do not use any form of rigid stick, pin, forceps or matchstick, etc.
- If the foreign body is not visible, ask the patient to blink briskly into a brimming glassful of clean water.
- Another method for removing invisible foreign body is to pull the upper and lower eyelids forwards and suddenly let go the eyelids. Try this two or three times and the consequent overflow of tears washes out the foreign body.

Foreign body in the ear:
- Gently pull the external ear towards you, to get a better view of the external passage.
- In the case of impacted seeds, slate pencil etc., do not put any water or oil inside as this will only swell the foreign body and make it difficult to remove.
- Do not use forceps, sticks or crochet needles as these can damage the skin inside the ear and cause infection apart from pushing the foreign body deeper inside.
- If it is confirmed that the foreign body is an insect, drop warm coconut/mustard oil or warm salt water into the ear with clean ink filler so that the insect either crawls out or floats up.
- In any case, a doctor's attention is necessary to avoid undue damage.

Foreign body in the nose:
- Make the patient breathe through the mouth and seek medical help.
- It is important to remember that any attempts to take it out worsens the situation.
- The nasal inner lining is more soft and delicate than that of the ear.

Foreign body in the throat:
- If the patient is gasping, nails and lips have turned blue, it is an emergency and needs urgent

medical attention to save his/her life. If the above stages are not present, then the following can be done.

- In case of an adult, make him/her stand and bend down forward.
- Approaching from behind bring both your arms forward and clasp the patient from behind at the level of the lower edge of the ribcage.
- Holding both your wrists together, make sure the knuckle of your hand is pressing the stomach area just below the ribcage arch in the front.
- At the count of three, suddenly pull your wrists into the patient's stomach. This sudden movement usually forcefully expels the foreign body out of the throat. You may repeat this procedure several times.
- In case of a child, bend the child across your knees and sharply thump his/her back in the hollow between the shoulder blades.
- Repeat this several times using your cupped hand for better transmission of the force of thumping.
- In the case of a very small child, hold him/her upside down by its legs and thump the back with cupped hands several times.
- In case of fish bones, thorns and open safety pins, the patient would have to be given medical attention. However, closed safety pins, round

coins, small marbles are usually passed right through the digestive tract and passed out in the stools the next day.
- Give several glasses of water to help in the passage of the coin, etc.
- If the lips turn blue and there is gasping, it means that the object has entered the breathing passage and medical attention is extremely urgent.

What is the First Aid for animal bites?

First Aid for animal and insect bites depend upon the animal or insect that has bitten it. Detailed below are the First Aid measures for common bites.

Dog bites
- It causes *rabies*, a disease that has no cure but can be prevented.
- All dog bites must be thoroughly washed with running water but the wound should never be rubbed or scrubbed, as this will push the virus deeper inside.
- The more the washing of the wound, the greater the amount of virus that will be washed away.
- Do not apply any form of carbolic acid, etc.
- Ensure that the patient receives the anti-rabies vaccine as early as possible.

Bee or wasp stings
- It can be extremely painful and the bitten spot may swell up.

- If many bees/wasps attack at once, the patient may go into shock.
- In the case of single bee sting, it should be remembered that the bee sting ends like a fish hook and cannot be simply pulled out without leaving a piece of sting behind.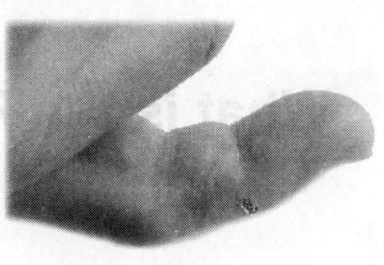
- The leftover piece of the sting can lead to infection and pus formation. Therefore, the bee sting should be gently teased out with the tip of a sterilised needle.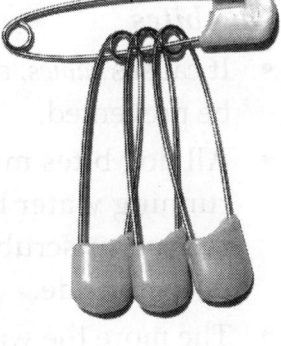
- A safety pin needle can be sterilised by passing it once or twice through the flame of a lit matchstick but make sure that it does not become red-hot.
- In the case of a wasp/hornet, the sting is not left behind in the wound, as it is needle shaped.
- In both cases, apply a weak solution of soda bicarbonate (baking soda) to neutralise the poison and reduce pain.

Scorpion bite

- Young infants and very old and sick persons with scorpion bites would need immediate medical attention as it may lead to a *shock*.
- However, in other cases, you can apply a weak solution of soda bicarbonate (baking soda) at the site of bite in order to neutralise the poison and reduce pain.

Snake bite

It is important to remember that all snake bites are not fatal and more people die from shock arising out of fear and terror than due to the poison. Steps for First Aid for snake bite include the following:

- Seek medical attention for antivenom injection immediately.
- Reassure the patient and try to keep him/her calm.
- Do not make him/her walk as this only pushes the poison faster through the veins. This is because while walking, the contracting leg muscles "milk" the veins.
- Apply a constrictive bandage on the 'heart side' of the bite in the case of bites on the limbs.
- You can make the constrictive bandage in an emergency by holding the two diagonal corners of a handkerchief and whirling it around to make a cord.

- Ensure that the bandage is firm enough to obstruct and stop the flow of the venom towards the heart.
- Release the bandage slightly and tighten it once again every ten minutes to prevent complete cut off of blood supply to the peripheral part of the limb.
- Do not cut the wound as this pushes the venom deeper into the tissues.
- Do not suck the wound as your mouth may have ulcers or cuts that you may not have noticed. The poison can harm you if it enters your blood through these ulcers or cuts.
- Gently wash and flush the wound thoroughly without scrubbing the wound.
- If breathing fails, carry on artificial respiration till medical help arrives.

What is the First Aid for poison?

Poisoning is a serious matter. You need to shift the patient to a hospital/or a doctor immediately with a note of the findings and, if possible, along with the name of the poison. Preserve packets or bottles which you suspect contained the poison and also any vomits, sputum, etc.

- In case the person who has consumed poison is **unconscious**, do not induce vomiting.
- Make him/her lie on his/her back on a hard, flat bed without any pillow and turn the head to one side.
- In this position, there will be no pressure on the stomach and the throat will be horizontal.
- As a result, the vomited matter will not get into the voice box and the tongue will not close the air passage. This is also the best posture for giving artificial respiration.

- Sometimes, when there is excess vomiting, the three-quarter prone posture — wherein the affected person is made to lie on his side with one leg stretched, the other bent at knee and thigh — will make things easier for the affected person.
- If breathing is very slow or has stopped, start artificial respiration and keep it up till the doctor comes.
- If the person who has consumed poison is **conscious,** induce vomiting by tickling the back of throat.
- Make him/her drink lukewarm water mixed with two tablespoons of common salt in one cup water.
- If the patient has consumed corrosive poison, do not induce vomiting even if he/she is conscious.
- Corrosives should be suspected if the lips, mouth and skin show grey, white or yellow patches. Acids, alkalis, etc., cause such burns.
- You need to dilute the poison by giving large quantities of cold water, preferably ice cold water. This will replace the fluid lost by vomiting.
- Tender coconut water is preferable to cold water as it contains nutrients and it also increases the frequency and volume of urine.
- The poison can therefore pass out of the body faster through urine.

- Give soothing drinks such as milk, egg beaten and mixed with water or *rava kanji*.

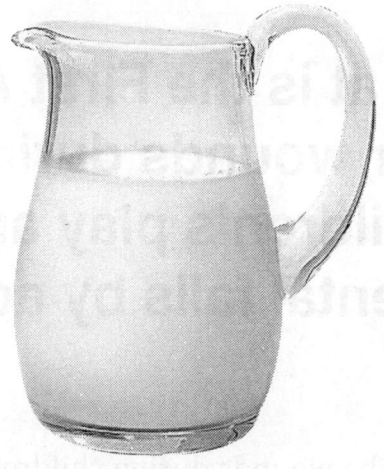

It is important to remember that delay in medical aid for poisoning cases always decreases the chance of recovery.

What is the First Aid for wounds during children's play and accidental falls by adults?

Most of the wounds during children's play and accidental falls by adults relate to scraping away of the skin. Such wounds, called abrasions, are very painful.

This is because the superficial nerve endings are partially damaged and therefore send out large amount of pain signals.

In case of a deep wound where the nerve endings are totally destroyed, pain signals cannot be generated.

- When the wounds open out of the skin, they allow dirt and germs to get in. As a result, you need to wash these wounds gently with clean water and soap.

- A soap solution made from pieces of soap agitated in a mug of water is preferable to using an actual soap.
- This is because the rubbing action of the soap can further damage the wound.
- Clean your own hands thoroughly with soap and water before washing the wound and do not wipe your hand dry.

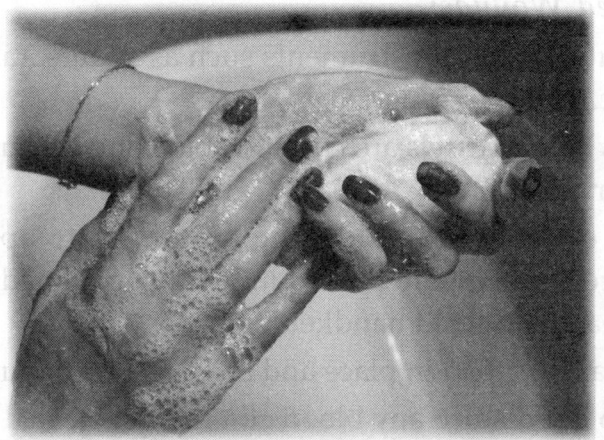

- Keep the wound only lightly covered. The naturally occurring scab heals this superficial wound.
- Do not remove the natural blood clot/scab because it is a protective seal on the wound.

Contused Wounds
- A hit by blunt object results in a contused wound.
- This is a collection of blood and damaged tissues under an unbroken skin.

- Since the skin is intact, a contused wound is a relatively clean wound.
- The accumulated blood sometimes presses against nerve endings and therefore causes pain and swelling.
- In such cases, put a handkerchief filled with crushed ice on the contused wound to relieve pain and swelling.

Incised Wounds:
- Cuts by sharp instruments such as a knife, razor, etc., cause *incised wounds*.
- As blood vessels are cut fully, bleeding is usually very heavy.
- In order to stop bleeding, you need to apply direct pressure to the wound with a pad made of clean laundered handkerchief.
- Leave the pad in place and bandage the wound.
- Do not disturb any blood clot that has sealed the cut.

Punctured Wounds:
- Stabs by knives, compass points, rods, etc., and bullet injuries cause *punctured wounds* which have a very small opening, but are very deep and could have damaged underlying organs, blood vessels, etc.
- Although the bleeding might be minimal in punctured wounds, this is the most dangerous

type of wound and requires immediate medial attention.

- Do not attempt to pull out the stabbing knife, rod, etc., since in their current position, they may still be "plugging" the cut deep inside the wound and thereby preventing bleeding.
- Pulling them out in the absence of surgical facilities would result in a massive internal bleeding that could prove fatal.
- However, minor pin or needle pricks or superficial knife tip wounds may be treated in the same manner as incised wounds.

What is the First Aid for a cramp?

A cramp is an involuntary contraction of a muscle. This may happen during exercise or by chilling. It may also occur due to loss of water from the body such as in cholera, excessive vomiting, excessive exposure to heat, etc. The muscles of the calf of the legs, hands, feet or thighs may get cramped.

Steps in management of cramps include the following:
1. Stretch the shortened muscle as follows:
    - In case of cramp in the calf muscles, straighten the knees with your hands and draw the foot up towards the shin.
    - You can also straighten the toes and make the patient stand on the ball of his/her foot.
    - In case of a cramp in the hand, straighten out the fingers with gentle force.
    - In case of a cramp in the foot, stretch/pull the toes towards the shin.

2. Massage the affected part and apply warmth.
3. If there has been loss of water from the body, give salt water.
4. You can prepare salt water by adding one teaspoon to one tumbler of water.

What is the First Aid for winding?

Winding results from a blow on the abdomen. The affected person may collapse because the *solar plexus* is affected. Solar plexus is the part of the autonomous nervous system that lies behind the stomach. Steps in management of winding include the following:

- Make the affected person lie flat.
- Loosen all clothing.
- Draw up his/her knees and thighs and gently massage the abdomen.

What is the First Aid for stitch?

Stitch is the term used for painful spasm of the diaphragm.

The diaphragm is the dome-shaped partition that separates the chest and the abdomen. It is made up of muscles and fibres.

A stitch normally happens during games and running. Steps in management of a stitch include:
- Rest the patient
- Give him/her sips of hot water
- Gently rub the affected side at the back.

What is the First Aid for heat stroke?

Heat stroke is a potentially dangerous condition that comes on suddenly and can lead to death if not medically treated. It occurs during very hot and humid conditions — both outdoors and indoors.

A heat stroke causes rapid failure of the temperature control centre in the brain. The person may become unconscious suddenly and his body temperature can rise very rapidly, i.e., up to 106°F and beyond while his skin would be hot and dry.

In this case, the body temperature has to be brought down very rapidly by removing all his clothes and sprinkling ice cold water on his body with a fan running to cause rapid evaporation and cooling.

Maintain the body temperature just above the normal temperature and call for medical help. When unconscious or semiconscious, do not give any fluids orally as this may result in choking.

Heat exhaustion:
- This is much more common than heat stroke, but can lead to a heat stroke if not treated, especially in children and old people.
- This is due to rapid evaporation of body fluids and salt through profuse sweating, but the loss can also occur in the absence of sweating such as in very dry places.
- The symptoms develop gradually with severe headache, dizziness, nausea and vomiting followed by unconsciousness.
- The temperature may be normal or slightly high.
- If the patient is conscious, give him/her plenty of very diluted salt water.
- Keep him/her in a cool place.
- Look out for development of heat stroke.

What is the First Aid for fainting?

Fainting is very common and is caused due to reduced blood supply to the brain.

Most fainting episodes occur due to psychological fears, but it can also occur when children are made to stand for a long time without any body movement.

This is because standing for a long time without body movements can cause the blood to collect in the legs. Usually the body collapses suddenly.

- As soon as the person faints, get his/her head down as quickly as possible such as by laying him/her down.
- Allow for plenty of fresh air and ask the crowd if any, to disperse.
- Loosen his/her clothing and if conscious, give him/her some cold water.
- Usually, the person recovers uneventfully.
- However, if the fainting attacks occur very often or are accompanied by any type of pain and

sweating, a doctor needs to be urgently consulted.

It is important to remember that fainting spells can also mean diabetic coma, insulin overdose or even heart condition.

In case of fainting due to diabetes:
- All people with diabetes must carry an identifying card, preferably attached to a thin necklace.
- In such cases, if the patient faints or collapses, send for the doctor immediately.
- Fainting due to diabetes can be either due to excess of *insulin* wherein the amount of glucose in the blood decreases or less of insulin wherein the amount of glucose in the blood is excessive.
- In case of excess of insulin, the skin is very moist with plenty of sweating with shallow and quiet breathing.
- You need to manage excessive insulin by feeding the patient with glucose water, crushed sweets or spoonful of jam provided he/she has recovered consciousness to some extent.

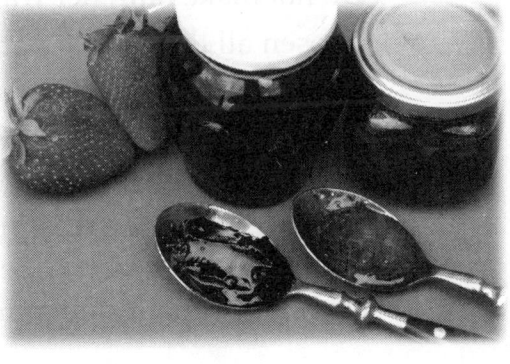

- In case of lack of insulin, diabetic coma can result. In such cases, you need to seek medical help urgently in order to administer correct dosage of insulin based on information from the patient's diabetic card hanging around the neck.

In case of fainting due to chest pain:
- This is potentially dangerous situation, especially in adults and older people.
- Chest pain may be due to an impending heart attack caused by lack of blood supply to the heart itself.
- If it were a heart attack, the patient would clutch his/her chest and collapse on the ground while his/her face would become very pale.
- There will also be profuse sweating.
- Nausea and vomiting may also occur.
- In case of a suspected heart attack, transport the patient immediately to a hospital without moving him/her unduly.
- Do not make him/her walk or sit up.
- Loosen all the clothing and give him/her lots of reassurance.
- Do not let him/her drink or eat.
- There is another form of heart attack, called *angina,* which also represents lack of blood supply to the heart. A person with angina may complain of pain similar to that described above.

- The pain, however, extends to the side of the left arm up to the little finger or upwards towards the throat and jaws.
- The pain is again very sharp. Management is the same as described for a suspected heart attack.

If the heart stops either due to suspected heart attack or angina, you need to carry out an external heart massage immediately within three to five minutes. Continue the massage till well after a pulse can be felt. It is better to always check the pulse as described earlier.

In case of fainting due to an epileptic attack:

- Contrary to old beliefs, do not attempt to put any metal objects in the hands of a person who is in the middle of an epileptic fit since the metal object can hurt the patient. This is because during an episode of epilepsy, the affected person's hands and limbs beat about in the uncontrolled convulsion.
- Do not hold down the hands or legs as the involuntary contractions can be extremely powerful and the resistance against your holding him/her down often results in muscle tendon or even bone fractures for the patient.
- Likewise, do not force the mouth open to insert any metal or wood piece between the teeth since it has been noticed that in many cases, the teeth of the patient have broken while biting down on the wooden piece.

- These loose teeth have been known to enter the air passage behind and cause choking.
- The epileptic fits do not kill the patient.
- Remove all objects around the patient as well as disperse the crowd around.
- The convulsions will stop by themselves and the patient will fall into a post epileptic sleep or drowsiness.
- He/she may act in a strange manner without his/her knowing till he/she fully recovers from the attack.
- He/she may even pass urine and motion during the attack.
- Keep watch over the patient till he/she recovers fully and insist on him/her seeing the doctor.

This is one situation where non-interference during the attack, is the best policy.

What is the First Aid for a fracture?

Fracture is the term used for an injury to the bones where there is discontinuity in the bone tissue. Most falls among children during play end up as wounds, but it is important to ensure that there is no fracture.

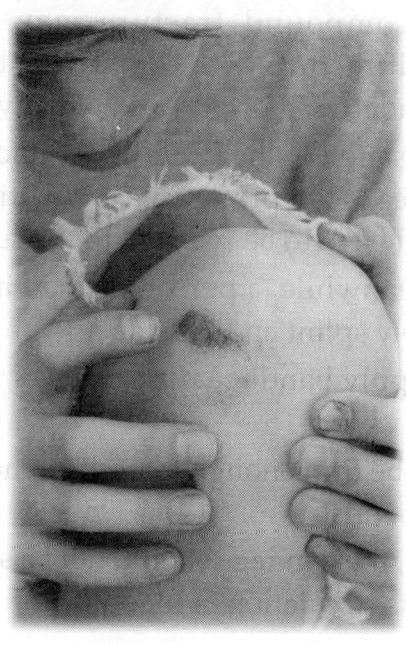

The signs of fracture would be a growing swelling over the injured bone. The affected bone is painful even on gentle touch, accompanied by a discolouration.

This is because of accumulation of blood under the skin. Often the child would refuse to even slightly move the fractured part. There could be a local deformity in the fractured limb.

Fractures can be simple, or compound. Simple fracture is the term used for an uncomplicated, closed fracture in which the bone does not break the skin. In a compound fracture, the broken end or ends of the bone tear through the skin.

Do not attempt to do any manipulation or reduction of the fractured bone. This is because a simple or compound fracture may become a complicated fracture with the broken bone piece rupturing underlying organs and blood vessels.

Immobilisation of the joints above and below the fractured area is the prime concern. Ultimately, all fractures will have to be referred to the surgeon.

In the meanwhile, a person trained in First Aid needs to apply splint and bandage.

- Do not apply bandage directly over the area of fracture.
- It should be firm enough to prevent movement of fractured ends.
- However, the bandage should not be so tight that it prevents circulation of blood.

- Padding material such as cotton, gauze or even folded handkerchiefs must be placed in the hollows of the body and between the prominent parts of the limbs.
- Do not lift the affected person to pass a bandage underneath him/her but use the natural hollows of the body to push the bandaged end to the opposite side.
- Bandage knots must be tied on the uninjured side only.
- Splints are used to support the injured limbs from bending and causing further damage.
- The splint can be any rigid piece of wood such as a foot ruler or even a steel ruler, or smooth pieces of split bamboo.
- The splints must be long enough to immobilise the joints above and below the fracture area.
- Always use cotton or soft cloth pads under the splints. Usually splints are applied over the clothing.

Fracture of the skull:
- Fracture of the skull may injure the brain, nervous system or the arteries and may cause concussion and compression
- Blood or brain fluid may flow from the ear, or nose, which may be swallowed and later, vomited.

- If the injury affects the bony socket of the eye, the eyes become blood-shot.

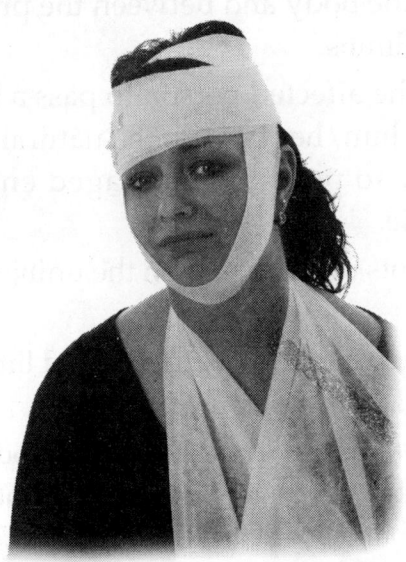

If breathing is soft and normal:
- Lay the affected person on his back with head and shoulders slightly raised by cushions.
- Turn the head to one side. If there is a bleeding from the ear, the head should be turned so that the bleeding side is down.

If breathing is noisy with bubbling of air through secretions in the chest:
- Lay the affected person in the three-quarter-prone position.
- Support him/her in this position by pads in front of the chest and draw up the affected person's upper knee.

- Keep the air passages clear.
- Do not give anything to drink.
- Do not rouse him/her.
- Maintain the same position in transport. Avoid disturbing the affected person.

Fracture of the lower jaw:
- This is normally the result of direct force. Usually one side is affected, but rarely both sides may be fractured. In most cases this fracture is a compound one.
- There is usually a wound inside the mouth also. The affected person is likely to have difficulty in speaking/opening mouth. His spittle can become blood stained.
- There is pain, which increases by speaking and swallowing. The face and lower jaw become swollen.
- The teeth look irregular and some teeth can fall. If there is an injury of the tongue, it may fall back and block the air-passage and there can be profuse bleeding.
- In order to provide First Aid to a person with fracture of the lower jaw, prevent him/her from speaking.
- Remove false teeth, if any. Make sure the tongue does not slip back.
- Ensure an open airway.

- With the patient leaning forward place the palm of your hand on the chin and gently press the lower jaw upwards against the upper jaw (which acts as splint).
- If the affected person shows signs of vomiting, remove your hand. Hold it in place again after vomiting stops.
- Move him/her to hospital. If the patient can sit, make him/her bend his head forward and downwards so that the tongue may not slip back and choke him/her.
- If the fracture is compound or extensive, turn the affected person's face down on a blanket.
- Next, place him/her on the stretcher with head projecting beyond the edge of stretcher and the forehead supported by hammock-like bandages tied to the handles of the stretcher.
- Place a blanket under the chest so that the head hangs forward.

Fracture of the ribs:

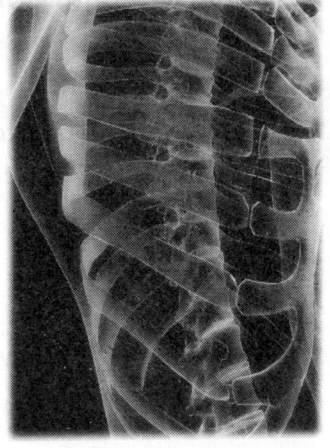

- This results in pain at the injured area. The pain increases by coughing and deep breathing.
- The affected person takes short, shallow

breaths so that the ribs do not move and increase the pain.
- If there is an open wound in the chest, the air is sucked in and blown out through the wound like the bellows. This is a serious condition and requires medical attention immediately.
- First Aid for a person with fracture of the ribs involves first making him/her lie down with raised head and shoulders and turned towards the injured side.
- Keep in position with a blanket folded lengthwise and tucked to the back of the affected person.
- Apply sling to the arm in the injured side. Transport by stretcher.

Fracture of the collarbone:
- The collarbone is normally broken when the person falls down on the tip of the shoulder or on the palm of the outstretched hand.
- The arm on the injured side looses partial movement. The affected person usually supports the injured arm at the elbow with the other hand.
- His head is inclined towards the injured side. The broken ends can be seen and felt.
- To provide First Aid to a person with fracture of the collarbone, support the arm of the injured side with the help of the affected person or an assistant.

- Do not remove the coat.
- Place a pad in the armpit.
- Leave the forearm free and bandage the upper arm to the side of the chest with a broad bandage.
- Support the upper limb in the triangular sling.
- Feel the pulse to make sure that circulation in the limb is free.
- You can transport the affected person even by walking, if his/her condition is not serious.

Fracture of the shoulderblade:

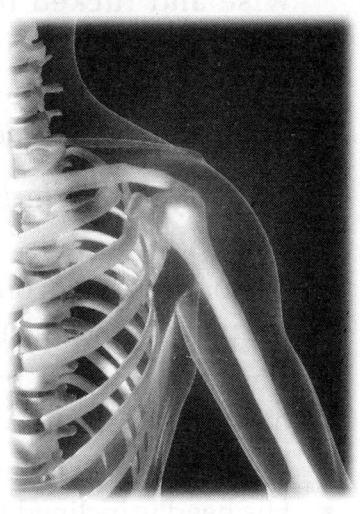

- This fracture is very rare and is caused by crushes and direct blows.
- In case of fracture of the shoulder blade, do not remove the affected person's coat or shirt.
- Support the limb on the injured side in a sling.
- Transport in a sitting posture unless there is shock.

Fractures of the arm-bone:
- This is a difficult fracture to treat as the muscles produce bends and overlapping of ends that are broken.

- Fractures can occur close to the shoulder, in the middle part, or near the elbow, including the elbow joint. First Aid will depend upon the part of the bone affected.

Fracture of the upper end of arm-bone:
- Place a pad of rolled handkerchief in the armpit and lightly tie the arm to the chest.
- Bend the elbow, place the hand on the opposite shoulder and apply a collar and cuff sling.

Fracture of middle part of the arm-bone:
- In this fracture, there is likelihood of shortening due to muscle pull.
- Stabilise the fracture by tying the arms to the chest wall — one bandage above and one below the fracture site.
- Support forearm in a sling.

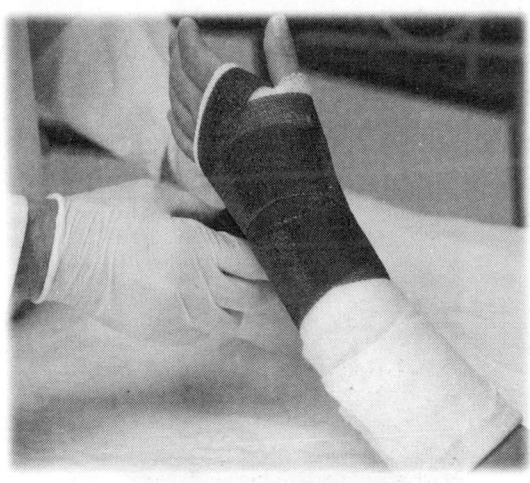

Fractures around the elbow:
- If the injured elbow can be bent, strap the arm to chest and support the forearm in a triangular sling.
- If the elbow cannot be bent, strap the arm and forearm by the side of body in extended position.

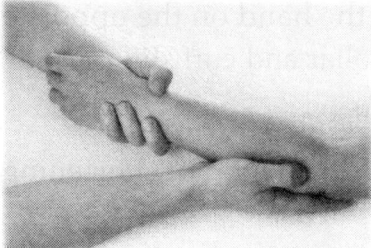

Fracture of the wrist:
- This is a very common type of fracture and is due to indirect force caused by fall on the outstretched hand.
- Care must be taken not to mistake it for a sprain of the wrist.
- There will be a considerable degree of deformity and swelling in a fracture.

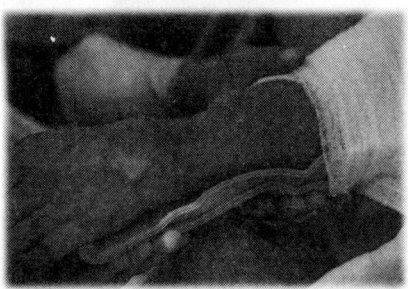

Splints in fractures of the forearm:
Forearm fractures are the only fractures where external splint is necessary. Steps include the following:
- Place the forearm at right angles to the upper arm, and place it across the chest, the thumb facing upwards and the palm over the chest.
- Roll a folded newspaper or other magazine round the forearm. The paper magazine should be from the elbow to the fingers.
- Apply one bandage above the fracture and the other over the wrist, first around it and then as a figure-of-eight including the wrist and hand.
- Support the limb by a broad arm sling.

Fracture of the thigh bone:
- This bone can break at any place along its length. Fracture of the thigh bone occurs quite frequently in old people because of small reasons like tripping.
- Do not take it for a bruise of the hip, but suspect a fracture. Fracture of the thigh bone is always serious because great shock results from it and there will be bleeding into the surrounding tissues.
- Healing is prolonged, especially in old people. Pain, swelling, shock and shortening of the limb can be noted.

- The foot on the injured side lies flat and turned to the outer side. The injured person may not be able to lift the foot to an upright position.
- To provide First Aid to a person with fracture of the thigh bone, immobilise the thigh by bandaging to the other limb up to just below the knee with padding between knees.
- If splint is easily available, apply a padded splint between the legs from the crotch to the foot.
- Tie the feet and ankles to the splint with a bandage.
- Apply a long padded splint from the armpit reaching up to the foot on the injured side.
- Apply seven broad bandages at the following places — (1) chest, (2) below the armpits, (3) pelvis at the level of hip joints, (4) both ankles and feet, (5) both thighs above and below the fracture.

Fracture of the kneecap:

- The kneecap can be broken by direct force; but usually the fracture is due to muscular force causing it to snap across into two bits.
- In this fracture, the limb is helpless as the important flexor muscle is out of action.
- There will be lots of swelling and bleeding. The gap between the two bits can often be felt.

Steps for providing First Aid to a person with fracture of the kneecap include the following:
- Lay the affected person flat with head and shoulders raised.
- Raise the injured limb to an easy position. This will relax the thigh muscles, which pull the upper half of the broken bone upwards.
- Tie to sound limb from thigh to below knee with padding between knees.
- Apply a padded splint from the buttocks to beyond the heel.
- Raise the ankle from the splint by pads.
- Apply a broad bandage around the upper part of the thigh.
- Apply a narrow bandage around with its centre on the upper fractured piece, cross it behind the knee and bring it up over the lower fractured bit and tie it off.
- During transportation the limb should be kept raised on a box, blanket or similar material.

Fracture of the leg:
- This is due to direct force, except when the lower part of thin bone of the leg is involved. There are two bones in the leg. Either one or both the bones may be broken.
- If both the bones are broken, all signs of fracture such as pain, swelling, deformity, shock, etc., are present. But when only the thin bone is broken,

no deformity is visible. This is because it is splinted by the larger bone. In case there is swelling around the ankles, you need to suspect fracture of the bones of the ankle.

Steps for providing First Aid to a person with fracture of the leg include the following:

- Tie the limb to the normal limb with suitable padding from thigh to ankle. Place pads between knees and ankles.
- Make a long well-padded splint and place it between the lower limbs extending from the fork to the feet.
- Without causing disturbance or pain bring the two limbs close to the splint.
- Place an additional pad between the ankle and knee and tie the feet and ankles with a figure-of-eight bandage.
- Place a broad bandage at the upper part of the thighs.
- Apply a broad bandage on the knee.
- Finally, apply two bandages of required size, one above and one below the fracture. Naturally, the bandages should be tied on the injured side; and note that if the fracture is near the ankle, one bandage should be omitted.

Fracture of the bones of the foot and toes:
- This is caused by direct injury such as a crush injury or a wheel passing over the foot.

- Suspect fracture of the foot and toes when there is pain, swelling and loss of power.

First Aid for a person with fracture of the foot and toes *with a wound* include the following:

- Remove footwear, cut or remove socks.
- Treat the wound. Use the other foot as splint.
- Tie the feet and legs together below the knee with padding between ankles, feet and knee.
- Apply a padded splint reaching from the heel to the toe over the sole of the foot.
- Place the centre of a broad bandage over the foot.
- Cross the ends over the instep and carry them to the back of the ankle.

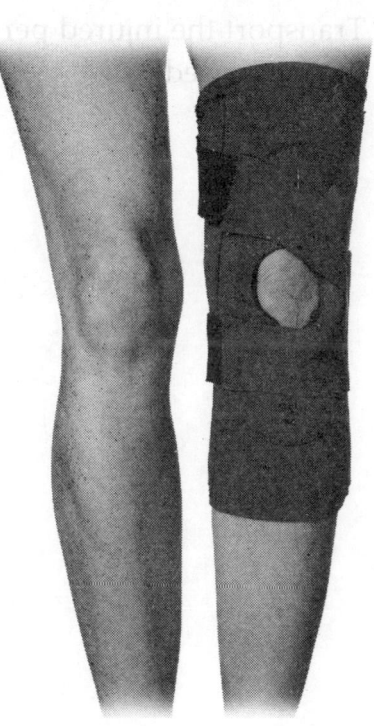

- Cross once more to bring them to the front of the ankle.
- Cross once more to bring the ends on the back of the ankle and tie it off.
- Raise the foot to make the affected person feel comfortable.

If *no wound is present* or suspected and if the affected person wears shoes, do not remove them, secure as described above with a broad bandage and keep foot raised to a comfortable position.

In case the injured person is not wearing shoes, provide First Aid just as you would for a crushed foot.

- Transport the injured person in a stretcher with the foot raised.

Recommended Contents of a First Aid Box

- Broad bandages
- Packet of blades
- Narrow bandages
- Roll of string
- Roll of plaster
- Bottle of Cetavalon
- Scissors
- Roll of cotton wool
- Forceps (blunt and sharp ended)
- One torch
- Packet of safety pins
- One strip of Paracetamol tablets
- Tube of antiseptic (Povidone)
- One set of wooden splints
- Tube of ear ointment (Gentamycin)
- Notebook and pencil
- Tube of eye ointment (Gentamycin)
- Small hand towel and soap

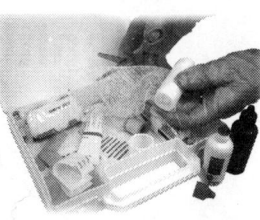

Health Solutions

ANXIETY
DIABETES
FIRST AID
HEART ATTACK
HIV/AIDS
MENOPAUSE
MENSTRUAL IRREGULARITIES
NUTRITION